Mediterranean Diet: A Clear Guide To Lose Weight & Increase Energy With This Heart Healthy Diet

by David Corr

This document is geared towards providing exact and reliable information in regards to the topic and issue covered. The publication is sold with the idea that the publisher is not required to render accounting, officially permitted, or otherwise, qualified services. If advice is necessary, legal or professional, a practiced individual in the profession should be ordered.

- From a Declaration of Principles which was accepted and approved equally by a Committee of the American Bar Association and a Committee of Publishers and Associations.

The information provided herein is stated to be truthful and consistent, in that any liability, in terms of inattention or otherwise, by any usage or abuse of any policies, processes, or directions contained within is the solitary and utter responsibility of the recipient reader. Under no circumstances will any legal responsibility or blame be held

Table of Contents

Introduction

Okay, so the word "diet" terrifies us all, right? Isn't it true? No one wants to go on a diet. No one wants to think about having to shed undesired pounds. No one wants to hear the words suggesting he or she needs to go on a diet. The word "diet" seemingly has remarkable powers, making even the most food-controlled-regimen-savvy of us cringe as it stirs up the notion of self-imposed restrictions, hunger, starvation, and deprivation. To the average dieter, the notion of dieting is a simple formula: *Dieting equals suffering*.

The truth is the term "dieting," is associated with the Old French term *diete* meaning, "fare or pittance," which certainly suggests the potential for self-deprivation, but the word is also rooted in words like *diaeta*, and the Greek *diaita*, meaning "dwelling, regimen, way of life," and "prescribed way of life." (Harper, 2001). The Mediterranean Diet is, in no way or by any means, associated with deprivation. The food included in the plan comes from every one of the existing food groups, with leniency placed on the red meat groups and some of the grains. With the Mediterranean Diet, you are never forcing yourself to starve or suffer from deprivation; instead, you are moderating intake of specified food groups and expanding the delicious possibilities you can put on your plate. Instead of viewing the Mediterranean Diet as another attempt to strictly control what you consume, you will soon begin to see how the regimen actually diversifies what you eat to such an extent you cannot possibly feel deprived!

The foods in the Mediterranean Diet are those common in Greek, Moroccan, Italian, Spanish, and French cultures. Many of the foods you have come to love will still be something you can consume, and you will be surprised at the great diversity you get from fresh foods, fruits, veggies, and seafood selections, with the occasional mix of lean red meats, legumes, nuts, olive oil, and red wine in moderation. Once you see the effects the diet has on the body and mind, you will never go back to eating another way – the Mediterranean Diet is not only healthy, but it works, and you will find you can carve off those excess pounds quickly. Best of all when you start looking and feeling good, your confidence will soar – this makes the diet a complete mind and body improvement regimen.

Many experts consider the Mediterranean Diet as *"The Heart Healthy Diet,"* including experts from the Mayo Clinic. In a recent article by Laura Donnelly, appearing in The Telegraph, Professor Giovanni de Gaetano also points to the diet as one providing considerable health benefits. The professor is actually the head of the Epidemiology and Prevention Department at the Italy-based IRCCS Neuromed Institute. In the article entitled, "Mediterranean diet better for the heart than taking statins, major study suggests," Professor Gaetano explains how the Mediterranean weight loss control plan is one well understood to promote exceptional nutritional intake and that those who adhere to the plan minimize the risks of chronic disease development.

Chapter 1: Defining the Mediterranean Diet

The Mediterranean Diet is a modernized dieting regimen that helps individuals lose weight while simultaneously learning how to make wiser, healthier food choices. The plan is one consisting of a mixture of cultural cuisines and tastes, including those from Spain, Greece, and Southern Italy. Unlike the Atkins' Diet where the dieter consumes foods approved for a high protein, super low carbohydrate eating plan, The Mediterranean Diet puts a focus on the consumption of very little meat. Instead, the diet promotes the high consumption of different types of fish, some dairy products (including both yogurt and cheeses), and wine in moderate portions, if desired. Additional allowances on the diet include a high amount of vegetables, fruits, legumes, unrefined cereals, and olive oil.

A Basic Mediterranean Diet Breakdown

One must bear in mind that a "full-fledged" Mediterranean Diet is a bit harder to pin down than the diet plan promoting healthy eating and weight loss. As the American Heart Association notes, there are as many as 16 countries surrounding the waters in the Mediterranean Sea, and there is a considerable divergence in diet from

one country to another. ("Mediterranean diet,
Since the region of the Mediterranean consists c
divergences in the way of economic, ethnic, cultu
religious ideas and preferences, a genuine Mediter
diet is a lot harder to generalize.

Some food sources recommended in the modernized
Mediterranean Diet may not be in every single
Mediterranean culture; For example, in Northern Italy it is
common to use olive oil only as a salad topper and not as
a primary fat source and butter or lard is for when cooking
a variety of dishes. Nevertheless, the modernized diet
consists of some of the most basic and expected
components and food choices one would otherwise find in
any Mediterranean diet, no matter what culture, ethnicity,
or peoples are behind the offering of the dietary plan.
Such similar components appear in the table below for
comparison.

Food Types	Allowances and Restrictions
Restricted or Eliminated foods:	A dieter consumes sweets, processed meats, red meats, and eggs in very low portions.
Fish & Seafood	Fish, which replaces much of the meat disallowed on the diet and proves to be a chief source of fat for the dieter, is acceptable in moderately high amounts. Blue marine species are the most

	acceptable forms of fish.
Diary	Cheese is an exceptional addition to the plan as it gives the dieter a healthy protein-filled food source. Yogurt is a component of the diet: Particularly the low-fat variants with live bacteria cultures in them as they are good for balancing the gut bacteria and aiding digestive processes.
Fruits and Vegetables	Any fruits, particularly those high in antioxidants, are ideal for snacking on or for dessert while on the Mediterranean plan. Vegetables are a large part of this diet plan, with an emphasis on those that are leafy greens.
Olive Oil	Virgin Olive Oil provides the main source of dietary fat in this plan.
Cereals, legumes, and nuts	Whole grain cereals that are unrefined and unprocessed are part of the diet plan. Legumes and nuts (especially the unsalted varieties) are also exceptional food choices for the dieter following this weight loss plan.
Red Wine	In moderation if desired.

A Bit about Fats

The American Heart Association, while not entirely backing the Mediterranean Diet as "safe" for those with cardiovascular conditions, quickly points out that those who consume a Mediterranean Diet are consuming less saturated fat than those who consume the traditional American diet (Mediterranean diet, 2014). The organization explains how about 50 percent of the fat calories one consumes while on the diet plan, which comes from olive oil, is a Monounsaturated fat that does not have a negative effect on cholesterol levels in the way the consumption of saturated fats does. The organization also explains how there is fewer heart disease related disorders and deaths when comparing heart disease related deaths in the Mediterranean regions and the United States, but scientists are not yet sure if this is due to the diet alone or perhaps other factors in play, like lifestyle, exercise levels, social supports structures, genetics, and environmental factors.

The Mediterranean Diet's History

Most simply stated the Mediterranean Diet is not at all what you might first conclude is a weight loss/weight control plan. Rather, it is a grouping of some cultural tastes, preferences, culinary proclivities, and a mingling of healthy, culturally defined eating habits. The culturally defined practices and taste preferences, when grouped together is identifiable as Mediterranean cuisine. Broken down to its simplest of rules, the dieters who partake of the eating habits defined by the Mediterranean plan are encouraged to focus on consuming fresh foods, primarily vegetables and fruits, whole grain products, and olive oil.

For anyone who hates the thought of dieting or controlling food intake, the Mediterranean Diet is as close to you can come to a plan where you can lose weight without that restricted diet feel. The foods are easy to prepare, affordable, fresh, and delicious. There is no need to make special meals for other family members, friends, or guests in your home. When on the Mediterranean food plan everyone will find the food choices flavorful and appealing. You never have to announce you are on a diet and this allows you to remain social and engaging with your friends, family, and loved ones.

When striving for the greatest health, we often fall short; we set out to remain true to a diet and fail. After several attempts, we start praying for help or hope that some miracle diet aid will strip off the excess fat. We are bound and determined when a diet begins, but the minute we feel too restricted, punished, left out, or deprived we give up on our attempt at weight control. Our frustration and ease in which we give up are why the dieting industry brings in billions of dollars in revenue every year – because manufacturers of diet aids know their audience – they know our fears, hopes, desires, anxieties, and frustrations. When you give up on one product, they expect your fears and hopes will eventually lead you to another. This continues until we find ourselves saying, *"I don't understand it. I've tried everything and I just can't seem to lose weight!"* It is an emotional battle everyday for someone who is mildly overweight, not to even speak of what an obese person endures in the way of beat down motivation, a lack of self-love and self-respect, fear, and frustration.

Treating Obesity with the Mediterranean Plan

Thankfully, the Mediterranean diet gives people a real working alternative and weight loss approach. A balanced mix of nuts, whole grains, veggies, fruits (fresh only), seafood, olive oil and, if preferred, the occasional glass of wine makes the acceptable foods and beverage list easy to remember. Of course, the Mediterranean diet is not a free ticket out of responsibility – the dieter will still have to struggle with the act of avoiding any processed foods, frozen dinners, and fast food. The majority of the foods permitted on the Mediterranean plan are those that are fresh, meaning in season.

How your schedule affects dieting and meal planning – The "chaotic life with too much work, no time for rest" American attitude toward everyday living makes it hard to put freshly cooked meals on the table every day. With little time to spend on the self, let alone with loved ones and friends, the American diet, one that is unhealthy and rushed, leaves us consuming foods filled with undesirable preservatives, additives, sugars, artificial sweeteners, unhealthy fats, and processed or refined flour.

The typical American diet is wreaking havoc on the health of many. As per information on the State of Obesity website (Trust, Health, & Foundation, 2016), In four states in the US there is an obesity rating at greater than 35 percent, and just over 30 percent in 25 more states and all states in the Union feature a 20 percent obesity rating. Middle-aged adults between 40 and 59 years of age are the highest percentile of those suffering from obesity, whereas 38.5 percent of the elderly aged 60 and older are obese, and the youngest adult group, ranging in age from 29 to 39 having about 34.3 percent of the group presenting with obesity. The healthcare costs resulting from the obesity related issues are nothing short of staggering and are between $147 and$210 billion each year (A, 1997c). If there were ever a time for you, to embrace a diet that, not only contributes to weight loss and management, but re-teaches you the necessary *rituals* behind meaningful food selections and cooking, that time is now.

Surprisingly, there are often unspoken benefits from bringing the Mediterranean Diet into the personal or family eating plan. With its focus on fresh foods and cooked meals and its dieters who are encouraged to do away with the thought of eating frozen dinners and processed foods, the Mediterranean pattern of eating is demanding dieters to slow down. We are all too much in a hurry today to focus on our health or to spend time cooking wholesome meals. When we are on the run and dealing with day to day chaos between work, home, immediate family, kids (if we have them), paying bills, home maintenance, and our myriad other adult responsibilities, how can we possibly have time to whip up healthy meal after meal like some magical domestic goddess that might do Martha Stewart proud? With the Mediterranean Diet, dieters can make eating meals a *ritual* again, one worthy of the time spent planning and cooking meals.

Cooking is one of the ways to nourish the self and others, but then so is taking the time to eat together and socialize. With the modern Mediterranean Diet some dieters might do well to add the rule to stash the cell phone and other distracting elements so that people can once again eat fine foods, and savoring both the flavor of the sumptuous foods before them, all while appreciating the good company they keep.

Supporting Science Backing the Mediterranean Diet

The Mediterranean diet is a relatively easy plan to follow, and it usually takes but a few minor adjustments to the way you eat in order to begin adhering to the plan. The general premise of the plan is more fish, less red meat. The fish sources you choose should be those that have high levels of omega-3 fatty acids. The latter-mentioned fatty acid is an essential fatty acid your body requires for optimal health; however, it is not a substance that the human body creates naturally. Therefore, we rely on food sources only in order to intake the right amount of Omega 3 fatty acids, with fish like halibut, tuna, and salmon hosting higher concentrations of the polyunsaturated fatty acids (A, 1997b); additional sources of Omega 3 include krill, algae, nut oils, and other plant life. The fatty acid helps boost metabolic processes for speedier fat burning and weight loss while simultaneously affecting blood pressure and cholesterol levels in beneficial ways. According to the University of Maryland Medical Center (UMMC), Omega-3 fatty acids assist in all of the following:

- Cognitive process enhancement and brain function
- Nerve development, activity, and vision
- Normal growth development
- Reduction in issues related to arthritis, cancer, and cardiovascular conditions
- Reduction in issues related to other inflammatory conditions

The UMMC suggests the Mediterranean Diet as an excellent source of Omega 3 fatty acids and further suggests the diet has "a healthier balance between Omega 3 and Omega 6," (A, 1997),: Since many of the recommended foods on the plan already contain the essential fatty acids the body needs.

This diet does not force you to do away with all fats, and in fact encourages the moderate consumption of healthy fats, particularly of the monounsaturated and polyunsaturated fats. The monounsaturated fatty acids we need for our health are found in foods like avocados, nuts, peanut oil, canola oil, and olive oil, as per information the UMMC shares on its website (*14). The same website explains the natural benefits of consuming foods containing polyunsaturated fats derived from olive, sunflower, canola, safflower, soy, and corn oils. It helps in lowering Low-density lipoprotein cholesterol (LDL) levels that are otherwise well-known as the bad type of cholesterol because it is linked to a higher risk of cardiovascular disease onset. Thus, the oils you consume while partaking of the Mediterranean menu lead to a reduced risk of heart disease.

Several studies indicate strongly the health benefits associated with the Mediterranean Diet. For example, as much as five ounces of red wine is acceptable per day on this diet plan, and wine has some beneficial effects on the cardiovascular system. Likewise, there are studies documenting the potential reduction in issues related to the cardiovascular system overall. What is shocking is just how poorly the Western Diet compares to the Mediterranean food pattern of eating. In fact, according to an article appearing in a 2013 issue of *The New England Journal of Medicine* entitled, "Primary prevention of cardiovascular disease with a Mediterranean diet," R. Estruch and a team of researchers were conducting a study involving the examination of both the Mediterranean and Western diets. During the study the researchers, realizing the potentially negative health consequences stemming from the Western Diet, were themselves faced with a moral and ethical dilemma Estruch R, et al., 2016); those participants on the Western Diet during the study faced serious health disadvantages. Thus, the group conducting the trial ended the study before its anticipated conclusion.

While the above-mentioned study ended early due to ethical reasons, it was not before the Mediterranean Diet was marked as being a healthy dietary plan. Physicians and scientists from around the world are recommending the

Mediterranean Diet, not only because the plan is diverse in terms of the permissible foods, but for the impressive health advantages. The Mediterranean plan is one that has demonstrated benefits that can help in the prevention of myriad conditions including metabolic syndrome, Diabetes Type II, stroke, and cardiovascular issues. The same food plan can improve bone, heart, artery, and kidney health while also serving as a regimen providing the body with cancer-preventing nutrients.

As per information made available by the University of Maryland Medical Center, helping in the reduction of cardiovascular conditions and negative health consequences in relation to such conditions is just the beginning of the benefits one derives from the Mediterranean Diet. The diet is one that might lead to the stabilization of glucose levels in the blood and it holds the potential for reducing cholesterol and triglycerides (A, 1997). One study appearing in the 2013 Spring issue of *The Permanente Journal*, supports similar arguments.

In "Nutritional Update for Physicians: Plant-Based Diets," Dr. Philip J. Tuso, Mohamed H. Ismail, Benjamin P. Ha, and Carole Bartolotto explain the rich benefits of plant-based diet regimens such as the Mediterranean Diet. The authors collaboratively cite the cost effectiveness of the diet as well as the low-risk interventions that can be used for the reduction of cholesterol levels, the HbA1C in diabetics, blood pressure, and the individual's body mass index as being some of the many benefits of a plant-based food regimen (Tuso). The researchers continue with the amount of medication a person must rely on can sometimes be reduced in some cases and the mortality rates stemming from ischemic heart disease reduced as well. Much of what the researchers cite as being part of the healthy plant-based diet is in the Mediterranean diet plan, with the researchers recommending a limitation on processed carbohydrates, oils, fats, and animal products while consuming an increased amount of whole grains, seeds, legumes, beans, vegetables, and fruits. Such a plan is beneficial for, not just cardiovascular conditions, but lipid disorders, high blood pressures, Type 2 Diabetes, and dealing with obesity.

Chapter 2: The Mediterranean Diet and Your Health and Longevity

With the Mediterranean Diet, you are getting far more than your average weight loss plan. The health benefits you gain from participating in the plan are many. Researchers have dedicated a serious amount of time studying the short and long-term effects of the food plan; their findings reveal the advantages the diet offers in terms of preventing and minimizing the effects of cardiovascular conditions, diabetes, hypertension, high cholesterol, and cancer prevention, among other health-related issues.

While the Mediterranean Diet does not have a rigorous exercise plan associated with it, it is nevertheless a good idea to partake of some moderate exercise to amplify the weight-loss benefits you can derive from the diet plan. Walking, jogging, running, swimming, or other aerobic exercises, done in moderation, can help tone the body. Thus, the diet plan and moderate exercise will prove, over the course of time, to be a complete change in your lifestyle: A move to a healthier way of living overall.

Cardiovascular Conditions

A group of researchers headed up by Ramón Estruch, M.D., Ph.D., from the Department of Internal Medicine, in

Barcelona, Spain, explored the effects of the Mediterranean diet plan. He specializes in general medicine, internal medicine, cardiology, nutrition, and dietetics. Appearing in a 2013 issue of the "New England Journal of Medicine," an article entitled, "Primary Prevention of Cardiovascular Disease with a Mediterranean Diet," reveals the research team's findings following the exploration of the health enhancing benefits (or absence thereof) of the Mediterranean meal plan and dieting regimen.

In 2013, researchers studied 7447 subjects. The researchers made sure there was a small control group and each member within it was on a low-fat diet only. The remaining two groups were on the Mediterranean Diet, with one using additional olive oil and the members in the second group consumed the Mediterranean Diet plan with nuts. (Estruch R, et al., 2013). The researchers monitored the subjects for a five-year period while looking at pooled risks for strokes, heart attacks, hypertension, and death stemming from cardiovascular conditions.

The results are remarkable, suggesting a 30 percent reduction of risks of stroke, heart attack, and death combined for those who followed the Mediterranean Diet with Olive Oil and a 28 percent reduction in the same health issues with those consuming the Mediterranean and Nuts plan. The more detailed findings suggest the results were significant for males, and that male participants faced a reduced risk of stroke by as much as 39 percent if they were part of the Mediterranean dieting groups. For those participants that dropped out, there was an 11.3% drop out rate for the low-fat dieting group compared to the 4.9% drop out rate associated with the Mediterranean Dieting participants. What's more, the researchers examined the subgroups they found that those with issues related to obesity, lipid problems, and hypertension responded the best when on the Mediterranean food plan. It is important to note that with this study, not only were there no noticeable differences in mortality rates overall, but there were no notable effects for females in the reduction in cardiovascular risks.

Similar studies reveal the Mediterranean diet may offer advantages over just taking statins. In an article appearing in *The Telegraph* by Laura Donnelly entitled, "Mediterranean diet better for the heart than taking statins, major study suggests," (Donnelly, 2016), the idea that both the use of statins and partaking of the Mediterranean plan is the most beneficial path to treatment for those with heart conditions. Statins are a group of medications that help in lowering bad cholesterol and triglycerides, including medications like pitavastatin, simvastatin, rosuvastatin, pravastatin, lovastatin, fluvastatin, and atorvastatin; whereas medications like the latter have been found to reduce mortality rates by 18 percent, the Mediterranean diet reduces the mortality rate by 37 percent. Some researchers lay claim that the findings "were not directly comparable," but also recommend that implementing the diet into one's lifestyle and taking statins simultaneously could give the individual the maximum benefits of both solutions.

Treating Diabetes Type II

According to the American Diabetes Association (ADA), the Mediterranean pattern of eating is better than a low-fat meal plan in terms of weight loss and weight control. Finally, the ADA makes a point to identify important potential associations between a minimized risk for Parkinson's disease onset, depressions, and Alzheimer's disease in those who choose the Mediterranean pattern of eating. Meanwhile, it's also interesting to note that the ADA remarks on how the eating plan really shouldn't be called a diet, but rather a pattern of healthy lifestyle choices, since the term diet seemingly connotes short term changes and not a permanent, healthy change in one's eating habits ("The Mediterranean diet - what's the story?," 1995). The ADA points to a recent study that supports the argument that the Mediterranean plan is an exceptional low-fat diet alternative and that the pattern of eating is also ideal for those who have pre-diabetes. The Mediterranean plan is suitable for weight control, which can lead to greater control over blood sugar, cholesterol levels, and blood pressure.

The Mediterranean plan is more successful than low-carbohydrate or low-fat diets — studies have revealed the low-fat diets can end up in the dieter actually gaining weight. In fact, researchers conducted a series of studies comparing the typical, and often highly recommended low-fat diet and the results of dieters on the Mediterranean plan; not surprisingly, those participating in the Mediterranean food plan had lower glucose, blood pressure, and fat percentages than those who stuck to a diet consisting of low-fat selections. The reason the Mediterranean Diet is more successful than low-fat diet solutions is that the diet continues to incorporate healthy, good-for-you fats, which, in turn, reduce the appetite by evoking a sense of fullness after eating.

Since the Mediterranean diet is a plan also featuring high fiber content, this also helps in developing a sense of fullness, all while helping in improving the absorption of nutrients and the digestion of foods. High fiber even lowers blood sugar levels and contributes to the improvement of insulin levels. Too much insulin in one's system can lead to the body's inability to lose fat effectively. Thus, fats begin to store up in the body and increase one's body weight. The Mediterranean Diet has its fair share of high fiber content foods, including the leafy greens, fresh veggies, and whole grains you are encouraged to consume. Speaking of fresh fruits and other produce, the latter contain carotenoids called lutein that, are great for vision, but also for promoting fat loss.

Treating Metabolic Syndrome

The Mediterranean Diet may have positive effects on a condition known as Metabolic Syndrome: A condition that consists of a cluster or grouping of metabolic risk factors, that when combined, increase the likelihood that the individual will develop cardiovascular issues. Metabolic Syndrome is a diagnosis given to an individual that has any three or more of the below-listed criteria simultaneously at any given time ("About metabolic syndrome," 2016):

- ✓ Triglycerides in excess of 149 mg/dl
- ✓ Systolic blood pressure of 130 mm Hg or higher
- ✓ Diastolic blood pressure of 85 mm Hg or higher
- ✓ HDL cholesterol of 40 mg/dl or less in males, and 50 mg/dl or less in females
- ✓ Fasting blood sugar level of 100 mg/dl or higher
- ✓ Excess abdominal fat (circumference of waist of 40 inches or more in males and 35 inches or more in females)

The regular adherence to the Mediterranean Diet was the subject of a study to see its effects, if any, on those diagnosed with Metabolic Syndrome. The study was headed up by Jordi Salas-Salvadó, MD, Ph.D., from the Human Nutrition Unit, Biochemistry and Biotechnology Department at the *Institut d'Investigació Sanitària Pere Virgili* in Reus, Spain, and the results appeared in JAMA Internal Medicine in 2008 in an article entitled "Effect of a Mediterranean Diet Supplements with Nuts on Metabolic Syndrome Status." The research team collected information from over 1200 participants in a PREDIMED study lasting the period of a year to see whether the Mediterranean Diet plan could reverse, and therefore eradicate, the effects of Metabolic Syndrome or not. One group of individuals consumed the Mediterranean Diet with Olive Oil and the other consumed the diet plan with Nuts. The group consuming the diet and olive oil had a 6.7 percent decrease in the presence of metabolic syndrome and the group consuming the nuts while on the plan had a 13.7 percent reduction in the syndrome (Salas-Salvado J, et al., 2008). Thus, the study's findings concluded that the

Mediterranean diet plan could, indeed, eradicate Metabolic Syndrome.

Treating High Cholesterol

LDL cholesterol is "the bad" cholesterol that increases the likelihood of development heart disease; certain behaviors increase the amount of LDL cholesterol in the body including habits like smoking, but also disorders like metabolic syndrome, diabetes that goes unmanaged, and a Western diet containing foods high in trans fats. In contrast, researchers have found the Mediterranean Diet can help in reducing oxidized LDL cholesterol from the body.

In a study headed up by F. Monteserrat from the Lipids and Cardiovascular Epidemiology Unit at the *Institut Muncipal d'Investigació Mèdica*, in Barcelona, Spain, the effects of the Mediterranean Diet on Lipoprotein are examined. Appearing in 2007 on *Jama Internal Medicine* in an article entitled, "Effect of a Traditional Mediterranean Diet on Lipoprotein Oxidation." During a study spanning the course of three months and the participation of 372 people, researchers examined whether those on the Mediterranean diet were presenting with oxidative stress markers like oxidized LDL cholesterol. The same changes were examined in those who were partaking of a low-fat diet, but the findings of the study only revealed a decrease in the amount of oxidized LDL in those partaking of the Mediterranean plan, while there was little to no decrease in the oxidized LDL in those consuming a diet of low-fat

(Fitó et al., 2007). Ultimately, the Mediterranean food plan lowers LDL cholesterol levels and thereby serves as a major contributor to the prevention of cardiovascular disease onset.

Cognitive Enhancements

The healthy foods you consume on the Mediterranean Diet have demonstrated so many wonderful health benefits, and among those benefits are some significant note-worthy cognitive enhancements. For instance, in a study appearing in the *JAMA Internal Medicine* in July 2015, entitled, "Mediterranean Diet and Age-Related Cognitive Decline: A Randomized Clinical Trial," researchers explain how the diet helps in minimizing one's risk of dementia onset. With vascular impairment and oxidative stress being two contributors to the decline of cognitive abilities as we age, they also serve as contributing to dementia onset.

Some epidemiologic research, however, has found the Mediterranean food plan, with its heart protective and immune system boosting features, has demonstrated the ability to delay or slow down the onset of dementia in the elderly (Valls-Pedret, 2015). The same study revealed an improvement in memory. Scientists are careful to caution that additional research is necessary, but that anything that can serve to delay the onset of cognitive deficiencies can serve as a tool for a longer quality of life in the elderly, even if a tool for total prevention has yet to be identified. So, what is it in the Mediterranean diet that helps in improving your cognitive health? The diet plan includes nuts and olive oil, both of which are cited as the source for counteracting the cognitive damages aging incites.

Just as the Mediterranean pattern of eating has dementia preventative benefits, in some studies it has demonstrated benefits in defense against Parkinson's disease. In an article appearing on the Parkinson's Disease Foundation website the connection between a reduced risk of Parkinson's Disease and the Mediterranean pattern of eating is explored. Parkinson's disease ranks second as one of the leading neurodegenerative diseases the elderly face, and researchers have found both genetic and environmental components to the potential onset of the disease and the speed of its progression. Since environmental factors contribute to the potential onset of the disease, various nutritional patterns and certain ways of eating, at least in theory, contribute to the onset or prevention of the disorder. According to the information in "Diet Affects Likelihood of Developing Parkinson's Disease," at least two studies have found specific patterns of eating demonstrate the ability to delay the onset or minimize the odds of getting Parkinson's (Foundation, 2012). One large study, in particular, cited the Mediterranean diet as a means of lowering the risk one has on getting Parkinson's disease, and a New York-based study revealed that those who do not partake of the Mediterranean food plan demonstrated an earlier onset of the disease. Essentially, the Mediterranean diet falls under the classification of "a protective diet," one that helps in preventing some neurodegenerative diseases like Parkinson's.

As per information Dr. Glenn Smith shares on the MayoClinic website, many studies on the Mediterranean food plan demonstrate positive cognitive effects. Not only does the disease so the potential to hinder the onset of diseases like dementia and Parkinson's, but researchers suggest it can help in the prevention of Alzheimer's onset as well. The myriad cognitive benefits the consumption of this healthy diet plan offer include memory enhancement, slowing of cognitive decline in the elderly, and it also reduces the chances one faces of dealing with mild cognitive impairment (MCI), the stage between normal cognitive decline and more grave conditions like dementia, Parkinson's, and Alzheimer's (M. Foundation, Education, & Smith, 2015). Smith explains how experts speculate the healthy lifestyle the Mediterranean plan consists of and the implementation of the plan improves blood sugar levels, lowers cholesterol, improves vascular health, and, in turn, minimizes risks related to MCI and the onset of other neurodegenerative conditions.

Cancer Defenses

In an article appearing on the Harvard Health Blog by Daniel Pendick, the former editor of *Harvard Men's Health Watch*, the author discusses a recent study revealing how the Mediterranean diet may actually help in breast cancer prevention, while also mentioning other health benefits of the food plan. Pendick points to a study appearing in *JAMA*

Internal Medicine revealing how older females residing in Spain and who adhered to the food plan and used olive oil were less frequently given a breast cancer diagnosis. The study involved tracking some 4300 females age 60 to 80. Of all the women tracked, 35 women were diagnosed with the disease. Of the females consuming a diet containing olive oil, there was a 62 percent decrease in cancer diagnoses (Pendick, 2015). While a healthy diet proving a preventative measure against breast cancer onset is no surprise, the study reveals those who consume foods based on the Mediterranean food pattern are also 30 percent less likely to develop strokes and heart conditions.

With all the fresh veggies and fruit in the Mediterranean plan, it should be no surprise the diet is effective and perhaps preventative against certain types of cancer. The fruits and vegetables are rich in antioxidants, which, in turn, serve as a natural defense against free radicals in the body. Free radicals can cause significant damage to the DNA in each cell and this damage can eventually lead to cancerous conditions. A diet rich in antioxidants is, for the most part, beneficial as it offers some natural cancer defenses through the foods one consumes.

IMPORTANT NOTE: Some research on antioxidants and cancer prevention suggest that the effect of antioxidants is only healthy for those who do not already have precancerous or existing cancer cells in the body; in such cases, antioxidants might trigger the release of p53, a "key tumor-suppressing protein." While it seems counter-intuitive to think the suppression of a tumor protein can prove detrimental to one's health, with the suppression of p53 is, it causes cancer cells to go unnoticed and therefore the cells "escape detection." (Thompson, 2014). Experts suggest anyone who has small tumors in the lungs or the potential for lung cancer, such as smokers, should be careful in considering the increase of antioxidants in one's diet.

The Mediterranean Diet for the Gluten and Dairy Sensitive

For those who might be gluten or dairy sensitive, the Mediterranean Diet is one that can be tweaked to accommodate your special dietary needs. For example, the Mediterranean diet puts a limit on the consumption of some dairy products, and this is great for those with dairy sensitivities. If you want to consume yogurt, which is permissible on the diet, but you are looking for a dairy alternative, opt for a soy-based yogurt product. If you are looking for milk to add to the whole grain cereal selections, you can opt for almond milk in unsweetened form. For those who are gluten sensitive, again this diet is something that can accommodate special dietary requirements. Rather than consuming barley, rye, or wheat grains, you can replace them with millet, buckwheat, amaranth, quinoa, and brown rice selections. It only takes a bit of creativity to make the Mediterranean Diet meet your unique dietary needs.

A Simple, Yet Effective Weight Loss Plan

The only way you are going to be successful on a diet is if the diet allows for three things:

1. A diet plan promising success must allow you to eat delicious foods and every meal and/or snack needs to prove appealing to the taste. Of course, the food sources you consume will also need to satisfy the body's demand for nutrients.
2. The diet needs to provide you with food sources that will give you a sense of fullness.
3. The diet that promises future success is one in which you do not feel deprived for following the plan – Being on a diet doesn't mean you have to starve.

If you end up with an eating plan that meets the above criteria, you are far more likely to experience success when it comes to weight maintenance, management, or loss. The Mediterranean plan meets the criteria listed above, and if you decide to change your lifestyle to improve your well-being overall, the Mediterranean plan is a system you can rely on to help you become the healthiest you can become!

The simplicity of this regimen is what makes it so appealing. There are not a hundred different rules to remember and no long lists of restricted foods. Even better, you do not have to pay for costly supplements or diet aids. A simple grocery list has you shopping for the fresh foods, lean meats, fish, and other ingredients. You do not have to worry about having to shop a lot for special or hard to find ingredients. When you can avoid some of the major pitfalls so many other dieters face, you already have an edge and a key you can use to open the doors to weight loss success.

What is great about the Mediterranean Diet is that many of the foods are not just healthy for you, but affordable. If you garden, you can consume fresh grown produce at very little expense, but even if you do not garden, there is always affordable, fresh, in-season produce available at farmer's markets, fruit, and veggie stands, and the local grocery stores in your area. When you begin to adhere to this diet, you will soon discover how it helps you lose and control your weight. As mentioned earlier, the diet plan allows you to slow down, take your time cooking and dining. This diet encourages socialization while eating, and can even help in bringing the family back together around the kitchen table to enjoy all of the fantastic recipes. The plan has some recipes that are equally adaptable for people on the move, as you will find when you explore the recipes shared in later chapters.

The Mediterranean Diet lends to fast weight loss because of the elimination of greasy, high calorie, low nutrient, processed foods and the replacement with far more delicious versions of your favorite foods in fresh form. You are doing away with chemicals, dyes, many preservatives, and additives, as well as unnecessary sugars and fats – but you will not miss a thing! Even better, you will not find yourself calculating calories on the go or counting carbohydrates and fats. All you have to do is eat in moderation, several small meals and snacks a day and eat foods from the Mediterranean list of cuisine choices. By eating smaller meals more frequently, your metabolic rate will improve and begin to help you in burning calories.

Chapter 3: Beginning the Plan

As mentioned earlier, being on the Mediterranean plan is considerably easy. Nevertheless, you may benefit from preparing in advance so you have everything you need at home to make the delicious, fresh foods the plan suggests you to consume. Consider this a time to clean out the refrigerator, cabinets, and the pantry so you can stock all areas with the wonderful foods you will incorporate into your daily eating habits. Not to worry, though, you are not expected to spend a fortune on special food products, dietary supplements, or any membership fees for assistance through a specifically established dieting community. You will want to make sure you have enough food at home so that you do not have to run to the store all the time: This saves you time and money as you can avoid impulse buys when you shop. There's no reason to rush the preparation process; you can take as much time or as little time as you might need to get ready for your new approach to eating healthy.

The Mediterranean Diet: Planning in Advance

Mark a date on the calendar that indicates the day you want to have the Mediterranean diet fully incorporated into your lifestyle. In other words, give yourself two to four weeks to work your way into the plan gradually. You can do this by writing down all the processed and frozen foods you plan to eliminate from your food plan. Clear that food out of your home and gradually eat less and less of the foods you want to do away with over the two to four week period. Things you will want to start eliminating include fast food meals, frozen dinners, excessive amounts of bread, chips, and empty calorie snacks. You should also slowly stop consuming cream-based soups and sauces. Below is a fast list of some of the foods you can start cutting out of your daily food regimen:

> Butter
> Chips
> Fast foods
> Bread (excessive amounts of)
> Cream-based soup
> Cream-based sauces
> Frozen foods
> Prepared boxed dinners
> Coffee/Tea with excessive sugar and milk or cream
> Regular soda
> Cut back on red meats like lamb, steak, and pork

Take some time to do a bit of window-shopping before you begin your diet. The World Wide Web is an excellent place to start looking for Mediterranean Diet recipes. Get a binder or two and print out all the meals that appeal to you. Print out an image of each dish so you can see just how appetizing it is when it is cooked – the visual part of the meal is just as important as the flavor. Make a list of the common ingredients the recipes tend to have, including things like spices and garnishing, and put them on your shopping list for later. If you want to get fancy, you can create a personalized Mediterranean Diet cookbook with the recipe and a photograph of the meal after you have presented it on a plate for consumption: Doing this will encourage you to give extra attention to the visual appeal of the meal.

You can add star ratings to the diet and your own feedback under each meal, so you end up with a recipe book where you can quickly locate all your Mediterranean-style favorites! Turn the cookbook into a long-term product by enclosing every recipe in a plastic sheet to keep it protected and attractive. You might even begin by trying some of the delicious dishes shared in the last few chapters of this book. When you are ready to shop, search for veggies and fruits that are in season: This will ensure great flavor and lower costs. Stock up on spices, virgin olive oil, unsalted nuts, and the other ingredients you find in Mediterranean Diet recipes.

Some Hints to Secure Your Success

Even though the Mediterranean Diet is one of the most promising regimens in terms of dieting success, you can always benefit from some success tips to serve as a motivational boost and as a bit of encouragement. Here you will find some simple hints to make the likelihood of weight control and management more successful.

Socialize during your meal and make the meal visually appealing.

If you are eating alone, you are not as conscious of what you are eating, as you are when you are eating in the presence of others. Whenever possible, plan to eat with friends or family and this will help keep you in check in terms of how much you consume while simultaneously allowing you to benefit from the positive atmosphere good company generates. While you are at it, you should make every effort to make every meal impressive visually. Every dish is a mini work of art and you can walk away from the meal having found it more enjoyable because the food is visually appealing. At the same time, you will be able to impress all your friends and family with artfully and masterfully presented meals!

Remember it is all about presentation.

Presenting food in such a way that it looks as if a professional chef has come to serve you; now this is one way to curb caloric intake while upgrading the appearance of a recipe. Do not be afraid to pamper yourself, your friends, and your family. Break out the fine china and ritualize your eating habits once more. In other words, lay out a tablecloth, some placemats, cloth napkins, and put a lovely vase of flowers on the table. Consider candlelight in the evening, and put a fresh peppercorn grinder nearby a saltshaker filled with pink Himalayan salts. Layout the food with a skillful eye for beauty and top it off with a lovely garnish or two. Spoil yourself when you eat: This serves a dual purpose of taking your mind off eating, and allowing you to slow down so you can really experience the foods you are consuming.

Remember there is no rush whatsoever.

This step can be the most difficult, especially if you are used to eating at work, on the run, on the bus ride home, or grabbing a quick snack to go as you head out your front door. Again, the ritualization of eating foods needs to be a practicing we implement to slow down, savor, and thoroughly enjoy what we are eating. At the same time, do away with the television, the laptop, and your cell phone device when it is time for a meal. Your full focus needs to be on what you are eating and you do not want any distractions.

Mix it up and adapt it to make it your own.

Have you spotted a recipe or two that you want to tweak to perfection? Then why not make the change? If a strawberry smoothie is more appealing than one containing a berry mix, or if you like one species of fish but not the other, simply make the switch and enjoy. Do not be afraid to experiment with foods that are safe to consume of the Mediterranean food plan.

Chapter 4: Eating on the Mediterranean Diet

When consuming the Mediterranean diet you will not feel deprived. You can break down your meal plans so that you are consuming several small meals a day, and because you are dedicating more time to the ritualization of eating, you will feel full faster. There are some tips you can benefit from as far as eating and timing your meals: Pork, lamb, and beef are very limited and, as mentioned above, are treated like acceptable small side dishes only a couple times a month.

1. Make sure you eat several small meals a day: This keeps your metabolism going and you burn calories faster this way. It also keeps your body from slipping into "starvation mode," or thinking that you do not have enough food to process: This mode hinders the metabolic processes in the body. Eat breakfast, a snack between breakfast and lunch, lunch, a snack between lunch and dinner, dinner, and if you feel a need to, a small snack before bed. It seems like a lot, but the meals are small and it will keep your hunger at bay.

2. Consume at least eight glasses of water every day. Yes, you have heard this before and it is for good reason. The water not only keeps you hydrated, but it helps your metabolic processes. You burn calories faster when you are hydrated. Additionally, when you drink water, it helps clear your body of toxins while it curbs your hunger.

What Foods Can You Eat?

First, the Mediterranean plan rids your diet of starchy, high carb, empty calorie foods, and replaces it with fresh vegetables and fruits. Yes, you eat red meats, but only a few times every month, and your primary protein sources come from fresh fish and nuts. When cooking, butter is hardly ever used and olive oil serves as its replacement. You will also be doing away with the heavier types of creams and sauce toppings, which is replaced with lighter sauce toppings, clear soups, broths, tomato based toppings, and vinaigrettes.

When you do consume meat on the Mediterranean plan, you need to consider it anew: in other words, it is not the chief portion of your dish, but rather a smaller portion and much like a side dish. The primary proteins, again, come from fish and nuts, but when turning to the smaller portions of meats integrated from a Western diet, chicken and poultry are primary choices followed by white meat pork, lamb, and eggs over lean red meats.

Meats: Poultry is permissible in servings of two to five serving a week, whereas red meats are confined to about three to five servings a month
Pigeon, pheasant, duck, quail, game birds, chicken, and turkey are some of the choices you can add to your diet.

So, how many servings of each food group should you get daily of other food sources? Follow this simplified guide:

Eggs: Two eggs three to five times a week
Eggs are a good source of protein. Choose those that are organic and free of hormones.

Fats: Four to six servings every day
When using olive oil on this diet, make sure you rely on the virgin and extra virgin variant. The extra virgin will cost you more but you will get far more flavor from the product. The virgin olive oil is also good for you and retains some of the flavor that the virgin olive oil retains. If you opt for regular olive oil, you are losing nutrients like some of the important Omega 3 fatty acids your body needs.

Whole Grains: Three to Five Servings every day
White bread has processed white flour in its ingredients so you will want to cut this from your diet, but you can replace it with whole wheat or rye. Brown rice, barley, oats, and wheat are excellent replacements for your whole grain selections as well. If you opt for whole grain pasta remember you are benefiting from the whole grain but that pasta is still starchy and high in carbohydrates (which can elevate blood sugar levels), so keep all pasta consumption to a moderate degree. A bit of pasta with many veggies is far more appropriate when partaking of the Mediterranean eating pattern.

Fresh vegetables and fruits: Four servings or more every day
With the exception of corn and white potatoes, there really are no limits placed on veggies and fruits. Bear in mind that boiled foods tend to lose the nutrients your

body craves, so opt for fresh, raw, steamed, grilled, sautéed, poached, roasted, or baked selections.

Seafood and Fish: Three times weekly at least
Allowable fish and seafood selections include Cod, Cold Water Fish, Crab, Haddock, Lobster, Mackerel, Mussels, Oysters, Salmon, Sardines, Shellfish, and Shrimp.

Dairy: In small amounts and up to seven times a week
Consider some of the following selections like Greek yogurt because of its high protein content, Soy yogurt (dairy sensitive), and Cheeses (low fat). The milk is reserved for coffee and tea most often, and you can opt for skim or low-fat selections. Cheeses are for small snacks or are integrated in meals.

Wine: Red wine is permissible every day in specific quantities.
For females, five ounces of red wine daily is acceptable, and men can drink up to two five-ounce glasses every day. In lieu of wine, you can opt for purple and red fruits to get enough resveratrol in your diet.

It is easy to build your shopping list from the acceptable foods listed above. Make your list by writing down foods to find in the meat, dairy, fresh produce and freeze sections – this will make your shopping experience easier on you and you can therefore make a better effort to avoid junk food aisles.

Dining Out

When you choose to dine out, it might wonder how you can stick to the Mediterranean food plan. Wherever you decide to dine, it is not hard to find cuisine that is well suited to your diet. For example, any salad is likely to fit right into the plan, and you can ask for olive oil or light vinaigrette to top the dish. Instead of red meats, you can opt for any non-fried chicken dish (if it is cooked with the skin, you can remove it before eating it). When asked what beverages you desire, you can opt for diet soda, or you can simply ask for water, tea, or coffee. Use sweeteners instead of sugar to sweeten your beverages. You should also try to avoid appetizers rich in calories and carbohydrates, in particular those made of white bread. If your meal requires bread at all, opt for whole grain, wheat, or rye selections. You just have to begin thinking creatively and you will soon find you can adapt just about any cuisine to suit the Mediterranean way of eating.

Simple One-Day Meal Plan

Below is an example of a meal plan for one day. You can take any Mediterranean diet recipe or acceptable food selection and insert into the One Day Template. You can also design your plan to cover a week at a time: This makes it easier to make up your shopping list. You can also adjust the recommended time for meals to suit your personal schedule.

One-Day Template Menu

Breakfast
8:00 am - Super Fresh Fruit Variety, 1/2 cup orange juice, 1 cup coffee black, water

Snack
10:00 am - Baked Banana, Pineapple, and Cinnamon, 8 ounces milk

Lunch
12:00 pm - Cheesy Meat Filled Red Peppers, water

Snack
2:00 pm – ice water, 1 cup tea or coffee, Fruity Parfait with Honey and Oats, water

Dinner
4:00 pm - Spaghetti Squash and Vegetable Blend, 5 ounces red wine

Dessert
6:00 pm - Chilled and Fresh Italian Custard, water or 1 cup non-caffeinated tea or coffee

Recipes

Welcome to the recipes section of this book. From here on out, you will find a ton of delicious meals and snacks you can integrate into your healthy eating plan. Chapter five covers breakfast, chapter six covers lunch dishes, and you will find some tasty snacks in chapter seven. Chapter eight reveals some amazing dinners you are bound to enjoy, and Chapter nine reveals some equally amazing desserts.

~Bon appétit!~

Chapter: 5 Breakfasts

Easy Fruity Smoothie

When you have a crazy morning and no time to consume breakfast this can cause your whole day to slump in terms of metabolic processes later on – It is better to get in a quick, delicious smoothie that you can not only make fast but take in tow if you are heading out the door to start your day. This tasty treat is filled to the brim with protein of the low-fat variant and it will keep your energy levels high until it is time for your next meal. What's more, the fresh berries are chock full of antioxidants and vitamins that your body craves.

Ingredients (Makes 1 Serving)
- ½ cup Greek Yogurt – plain vanilla, low-fat variety
- ½ cup frozen or fresh strawberries, blueberries, or a mix of the berries of your choosing (*potential variations include raspberries, thimbleberries, or blackberries*)
- ¼ cup milk – low-fat or skim
- 10 full ice cubes or the crushed equivalent

Directions: Put the berries and yogurt in the blender and puree the mix. Add in the ice and milk and continue pureeing until the shake is an ultra smooth liquid. Enjoy!

Whole Grains and Fruit Breakfast

Fresh berries and whole grain oats give your body the right amount of fiber and you will absolutely love the taste of this quick and easy breakfast meal. The antioxidants in the berries are exceptional for destroying free radicals in the body, and the hefty doses of vitamin C serve as a natural boost to your immune functioning while helping in fending off free radicals in the body thanks to the antioxidants coming from this vitamin-rich breakfast. Better yet, with the consumption of all natural, unsalted walnuts, you are getting a bit of the metabolic boosting omega 3 fatty acids, not to mention the natural cognitive enhancements.

Ingredients (Makes 2 Servings)
- ½ cups of oats (quick cooking, non-instant, or whole grain rolled varieties)
- ¾ cups of blackberries, raspberries, blueberries, or all of the latter
- 2 teaspoons of pure, raw honey
- 2 tablespoons walnuts – pieces or crushed

Directions: Follow the instructions on the labeling of the oats in order to prepare them. Once cooked, add the oats to two dishes. Makes sure the dishes are deep enough to allow the addition of the berry mixture and remaining ingredients.

Put the berries, walnuts and honey in the microwave for half a minute. Top off oats with the mixture. Enjoy!

Healthy Frittata

If you like the flavor of a frittata, you'll appreciate this Healthy Frittata recipe, and if you are tired of throwing away small amounts of leftover veggies all the time, here's a recipe that will help you get the most out of your grocery bills.

Ingredients (Makes 8 Servings)
- ¼ sweet onion – diced
- ¼ teaspoon ground pepper – fresh
- ½ green pepper – diced
- ½ teaspoon of salt
- ½ yellow winter squash – diced
- 1 tablespoon chopped fresh parsley
- 1 tablespoon fresh basil – chopped
- 1 teaspoon extra virgin olive oil
- 6 to 8 cherry tomatoes – sliced in half
- 8 whole eggs – scrambled

Directions: Heat the extra virgin olive oil over medium heat in a large skillet; Add to the skilled the green bell peppers, sweet onions, and diced winter squash. Cook all ingredients until the onions become see through – this should take just under five minutes. Now add the parsley, basil and halved cherry tomatoes. Sprinkle with the fresh ground pepper and salt. Allow to cook for about 60 seconds and then pour in all of the scrambled eggs as you cover all the ingredients inside the skillet. Cover the skillet. Turn down the stove heat to low and let the dish cook about six minutes or until you have thoroughly cooked eggs. Once finished, put the frittata onto a plate or platter and cut up into slices.

Super Fresh Fruit Variety

Fruit salad seems like a staple of the summertime meal plans. With this delightful dish, you are mingling berries, melon, and a touch of coconut for a salad of amazing color and flavor. You can make this recipe quickly, without much fuss, and it will last a full three days in the fridge. Some inexpensive plastic containers with covers will allow you to tote some to work for lunch or snack, or just save a bit for an after dinner treat. It makes a great breakfast dish too.

Ingredients (Makes 8 Servings)
- ➢ 1 large lime – juice and zest
- ➢ 1 cup blueberries – fresh
- ➢ 1 cup strawberries – fresh and halved
- ➢ 1/2 coconut flakes – toasted and unsweetened

- ➢ 1/2 cup olive oil – extra virgin
- ➢ 1/4 honey – pure and raw
- ➢ 2 cups cantaloupe – cubed
- ➢ 2 cups honeydew – cubed
- ➢ 2 cups seedless grapes – red variety

Directions: *Salad:* In a big bowl, add the lime zest, coconut, and all the fresh fruit. Stir until well mixed. Set aside.

Dressing: In your blender, add the salt, juice of lime, and the pure honey. Blend well then add virgin olive oil slowly to the existing mix. The mixture should become opaque in appearance.

Drizzle the fresh dressing over the fruit mix salad. Chill for at least four hours and remix the salad before dishing out into attractive salad bowls.

Chapter: 6 Lunch

When it comes to lunch meals you want dishes that are quick to prepare. If you work during your lunch hour, bring a lunch sack with a helping of last night's dinner or make extra helpings to cover a few days time. This will allow you to continue to eat fresh while refraining from frozen meals.

Cheesy Meat Filled Red Peppers

This dish brings a variety of veggies together for a stuffed peppers recipe like no other. To visually dress up the dinner, opt for green and yellow or orange peppers too; the color splash will make the dish all the more visually delightful.

Ingredients (Makes 2 Servings)
- 4 red peppers – whole, large, firm, and ripe
- 1 can crushed tomatoes
- 2 cups whole grain rice
- 1 cup of sausage
- 1 tablespoon olive oil – extra virgin
- 2 garlic cloves – fresh and minced
- 1/2 fresh onion – yellow variant, diced
- 1/2 pound cremini or white sliced mushrooms
- 1 tablespoon basil – fresh, chopped
- 1 tablespoon oregano – chopped, fresh

- ➢   1/2 teaspoon salt
- ➢   1/4 black pepper – freshly ground
- ➢   1 cup mozzarella cheese – shredded and part-skim
- ➢   1 tablespoon Parmesan cheese – grated

Directions: Have the oven set to heat at 375 degrees Fahrenheit when preheating. Using a cookie sheet, line the pan with aluminum foil.

Take a slice off the top of each red pepper to open them up and to reveal the seeds inside. Remove all the seeds and interior of the peppers.

Cook the half cup of sausage and drain it. In a separate pan, boil the whole grain rice. Stir in the can of crushed tomatoes. Then in a separate pan, heat fresh virgin olive oil in a large skillet. Add oregano, basil, onions, mushrooms, and garlic. Sauté for about five minutes; add a touch of salt and pepper to taste.

Add the mozzarella cheese, rice, tomatoes, and sausage together in a bowl and mix well. Scoop the mix of veggies and spices in the skillet into the bowl with the other ingredients. Take the mix and fill each pepper back up to the top. Sprinkle with Parmesan. Bake in oven for 20 minutes or until the red peppers are tender.

Mild-Flavored Cajun Shrimp Salad

A wonderful lunch or side dish for dinner, this Cajun Shrimp Salad is simple to make and absolutely delicious. If you want to change it up a bit you can add a 1/2 can of tuna packed in water or toss in a few fresh scallops cooked in olive oil.

Ingredients (Makes two servings)
10 to 15 jumbo shrimp
- ➢ 2 cups butter lettuce – shredded
- ➢ 1/2 cup carrots – finely sliced
- ➢ 1/2 cup red cabbage –shredded
- ➢ 8 small cherry tomatoes – orange in color and halved
- ➢ 1 tablespoon Parmesan Cheese
- ➢ 4 tablespoons olive oil – divided
- ➢ 2 tablespoon Cajun spices - divided

Directions: Remove the shells and tails from the shrimp before cooking. Rinse the shrimp and place in a bowl, but allow the shrimp to remain wet following the rinse. In a small bowl, add the Cajun spices. Put two tablespoons of olive oil into the skillet and heat on medium-high. Add shrimp in the bowl with Cajun spices one by one and then place into the skillet in a single layer so all the shrimp can cook evenly.

Cook the shrimp thoroughly until the shrimp turns from a translucent gray color to a vibrant, fresh pink color. It takes about two to three minutes on each side to cook properly. Sprinkle the other tablespoon of Cajun spices over the shrimp. Allow shrimp to cool.

In a large bowl, add the lettuce, carrots, red cabbage, and halved cherry tomatoes. Top with cooked shrimp. Add two tablespoons olive oil for dressing and top with fresh Parmesan.

Mediterranean Lettuce and Lobster Wrap

Instead of overloading on hefty carbohydrates, you can do away with the bread you might need for a sandwich and use fresh, large leaves of lettuce as a healthy veggie wrap instead. Add ingredients, wrap, and enjoy!

Ingredients (Makes Two Serving)
- 1/2 cup fresh lobster meat
- Himalayan pink salt – just a pinch
- Freshly ground pepper –just a pinch
- 2 tablespoons of Mayo with olive oil or just straight olive oil for dressing
- 2 slices ripe tomato – each sliced in half down the middle to make for halved slices
- 4 large lettuce leaves
- 1/2 fresh basil – finely chopped
- 1/2 fresh parsley – finely chopped
- 2 small fresh lemon slices

➢ 2 tablespoons olive oil (4 tablespoons if you opt out on the Mayo)

Directions: In a large bowl, add Lobster, salt, pepper, Mayo or olive oil, basil, and parsley. Mix thoroughly.

On two separate plates layout two lettuce leaves; make one overlap the other so it creates a long enough wrap to enclose the ingredients. Splitting the mix in half, place it on the lettuce while forming about a two-inch thick line about two inches from the edge of the aligned lettuce. Squeeze a touch of lemon on each wrap.

Place two of the halved slices tomatoes to top of the mixture. Add olive oil for topping if you decided not to use Mayo. Wrap the lettuce tightly around the ingredients. Enjoy!

Chapter 7: Snack

Quick and Tasty Cucumber Sandwiches

For when you are in need of a fast snack, you can raid the fridge in a healthy way. This snack takes mere minutes to make and will hold you over until dinnertime. What's more, you will gain the added benefit of keeping your metabolic processes in check.

Ingredients (Makes Two Servings)
1 – large, fresh cucumber
1 – can of tuna packed in water
1 – stalk of celery – finely diced
2 slices of pepper jack cheese
Two tablespoons of Mayo with Olive Oil

Directions: Slice up the cucumber into 1/2 slices. Count out an even amount of slices, with each sandwich consisting of two cucumber slices. Set aside. Chop up the stalk of celery into tiny pieces. Drain the water from the tuna, mix in the celery, and add the two tablespoons of Olive Oil Mayo. Cut the pepper jack slices into small one-inch squares. Take a cucumber slice and top it with the cheese, tuna mix, and a second cucumber slice. Serve immediately.

Baked Banana, Pineapple, and Cinnamon

There's nothing like some of your favorite fruit to keep you going during that mid-afternoon energy slump. This recipe has all the right ingredients to keep you satisfied. You can also consider swapping out the banana slices for apples or pears.

Ingredients (Makes Six Servings)
- 1 – large pineapple – peeled and cut into round slices
- 2 – large bananas – peeled and cut into 1/2 slices
- Cinnamon
- 2 tablespoons of pure, raw unprocessed honey
- 1 tablespoon Greek Yogurt

Directions: Preheat your oven to 325 degrees. Cut and peel the pineapple and cut into inch thick rings. Cut and peel the bananas and cut into 1/2 slices. Using two flat baking sheets, cover both with aluminum foil. Layout the pineapple on one pan and layer the bananas onto the other creating a flat layer with the banana pieces. Bake both for 8 to 10 minutes. Put a pineapple slice down onto a plate and top it with the baked bananas. Heat the honey in the microwave for about 30 seconds and stir in cinnamon. Use this mix to drizzle over the bananas and pineapple. Top off with another pineapple. Top that with a spoonful of vanilla Greek yogurt.

Fruity Parfait with Honey and Oats

Consuming whole grains is easy when you partake of this parfait for breakfast. You can store the nut and oats mixture for up to 14 days with an airtight plastic container and the mix is a simple, tasty snack if you happen to make extra. You can have this Parfait with a side of toast or cereal.

Ingredients (Makes 2 Serving)
- ➢ 1/2 cup whole-grain oats or quick cooking variants
- ➢ 1 teaspoon raw, unprocessed honey
- ➢ 1/2 cup walnut (crushed or in pieces)
- ➢ 1 cup strawberries – fresh and halved
- ➢ 1 1/2 cups vanilla Greek Yogurt – low-fat (about 12 ounces)
- ➢ Mint leaves

Directions: You will need to preheat the oven to 300 degrees Fahrenheit.
Put the walnuts and oats onto a baking sheet and spread out across the pan to create a flat layer. Allow the ingredients to toast in the oven up to 12 minutes. Pull from the oven and allow to cool.

Put the honey in a bowl in the microwave and heat it up until it is warm – this should take about a half a minute. Put strawberry halves into the warm honey and stir gently.

In two dessert bowls, put a small, thin layer (about a tablespoon) of the strawberries and honey on the bottom of each bowl. Put yogurt on top of the fruit and honey and top off with the oat and nut mix. Continue adding ingredients in this manner and order until you reach the top of the dessert bowl or dish, which should be able to hold at least eight ounces. You can eat the dessert warm, or cool it for later consumption. Top off with fresh mint leaves as a garnish.

Banana & Strawberry Smoothie

Here is what you need when you have one foot already out the door in the morning in order to keep up with your chaotic schedule and personal plans. The Banana and Strawberry Smoothie is a perfect replacement for the sit-down type of meal. You get plenty of protein and good gut bacteria from the Greek Yogurt and the treat is easy to make. Fast to eat and filling, fresh, or frozen peaches work with this recipe.

Ingredients (Makes 2 Serving)
- 1 bananas, peeled and sliced
- 1 cup fresh strawberries, halved
- 6 ounces of Greek Yogurt – vanilla or strawberry for extra berry flavor
- 8 Ice Cubes

Directions: Put everything in the blender. Mix on high to pulverize ingredients. Best if served chilled and even better on crushed ice!

Chapter 8: Dinner

Dinner should be the most ritualized meal of the day; it is typically the time everyone gets home and eating dinner together is a great way to unwind. The best trigger for relaxation is a warm, hot, satisfying meal. Here you will find some dishes that will keep everyone in the family craving time at your dinner table.

Tortellini in Fresh Veggie Soup

Meat filled Tortellini in fresh vegetable soup; this dish makes or spectacular meal on a cold, cool night, or during the winter months when you want to warm up fast and savor some delicious food! Swap out the Tortellini with fresh cheese filled Ravioli, or simply use veggie noodles for a twist and to add a visually appealing dash of color to the dish! Make an extra batch and store it in the fridge if you have a busy week ahead and you can have extra for lunch or dinner the next day.

Ingredients (Makes about 4 Servings)
- 1 – 9-ounce package of meat filled Tortellini
- 1 can of vegetable broth (about 15 ounces)
- 1 clove fresh garlic – minced
- 1 cup yellow squash - diced
- 1 cup zucchini – diced
- 1 half cup fresh green pepper – chopped into small cubes

- 1 half cup fresh red pepper – chopped into small cubes
- 1 large tomato, ground up in food processor
- 1 tablespoon olive oil – extra virgin variety
- 1 teaspoon fresh basil
- 1 teaspoon fresh marjoram
- 1/2 cup fresh cut celery – chopped
- 1/2 cup hot water
- 1/4 cup fresh carrots – diced
- Pinch of fresh ground pepper (as preferred)
- Pinch of salt (as preferred)

Directions: In a large Dutch oven pan, cook the extra virgin olive oil over medium heat. Add green peppers, red peppers, carrots, celery, and fresh garlic. All the veggies to cook for roughly a minute before pouring the broth into the pan. Pour in the hot cup of water, the freshly crushed tomatoes, and the marjoram and basil. Cook until the mixture comes to a rolling boil.

Put the Tortellini into the mixture and allow them to cook for about five minutes less than the package suggests. This will then allow you to add the yellow squash and zucchini, and bring to a second boil. Allow to cook for three to five minutes more. Stir in a pinch of salt and pepper.

Spaghetti Squash and Vegetable Blend

If you want something loaded with veggies, this dish is perfect. You can also add some shrimp, scallops, or grilled chicken to mix up this recipe for something new. This is a terrific dish if you have a lot of leftover veggies from other recipes: You can toss in just about any vegetables so you are not wasting your produce.

Ingredients (Makes 4 Servings)
- ➤ 2 Spaghetti squash
- ➤ 2 cups cauliflower
- ➤ 2 cups Brussels sprouts
- ➤ 1 cup fresh spinach – finely chopped
- ➤ 1 cup carrots
- ➤ 1 cup peas
- ➤ 1 cup green beans
- ➤ 1/2 cup water
- ➤ 2 tablespoons parmesan
- ➤ 2 tablespoons Olive Oil
- ➤ Pinch of salt
- ➤ Pinch of pepper

Directions: Preheat your oven to 375 degrees. Cut each squash into halves lengthwise. Remove any of the seeds with a spoon. Put the spaghetti squash cut side down into a casserole dish measuring 9 x 13. Add 1/2 cup of water and allow the squash to bake for about 35 minutes until the interior is soft. Take a fork and move it back and forth over the surface of the squash; it should come apart into ribbons or strands and look like spaghetti noodles.

Put the carrots in the steamer basket and steam for four minutes. Then add the broccoli, green beans, and cauliflower in the steamer basket and steam for another four minutes. Add the spinach and peas and steam for an additional three minutes until all veggies are tender.

Put the spaghetti squash into bowls and top with steamed veggies. Drizzle Olive Oil over the top and add a touch of parmesan. Season with salt and pepper to taste.

Oven Roasted Haddock with Lemon

For a light dinner that is sure to satisfy, give this roasted Haddock recipe a try. If you prefer, you can swap out the Haddock for flounder. You also have the option of breading the fish with Greek yogurt and a product like Bisquick®, but if you are looking to manage your weight, you might want to skip the breading entirely.

Ingredients (Makes 4 Servings)
- ½ teaspoon freshly chopped oregano
- ½ teaspoon of salt
- Fresh ground pepper to taste
- 1 ½ pounds of fresh Haddock fillets
- Four sprigs of parsley
- 1 cup of dill pickles (finely diced)
- 1 cup of Olive Oil Mayo
- 1 – lemon

Directions: Preheat the oven to 450 degrees. Prepare a cooking dish large enough to hold the pound and a half of Haddock laid out into long thick slices. Before putting the fresh fish into the dish, give the pan good coating of a non-stick spray. Lay fish into the pain and sprinkle with salt, fresh pepper, oregano, and squeeze some fresh lemon juice onto each piece before putting it into the oven.

Bake about 20 minutes until the fish is flaky, crisp, and tender: You can test the fish with a fork. While baking, mix the Mayo with Olive Oil with two tablespoons finely diced pickles to make relish. When the fish is finished, squeeze a touch of lemon over the fillets once more. Add parsley sprigs to the top of the fillets and serve with a side of homemade relish. Serve as is or with a side of veggies.

Veggie Dinner Omelet

Every once in a while, you just want a great breakfast meal for dinner. When you are looking for something quick and light. Put all the remaining veggies from other dishes you have made to use in this dish or pull out some that are fresh to the season.

Ingredients (Makes 2 Servings)
- ➢   2 tablespoons – olive oil (extra virgin and divided)
- ➢   1 freshly minced clove of garlic

- ➢ 1/2 thinly sliced red bell pepper
- ➢ 1/4 thinly sliced fresh red onion
- ➢ 2 tablespoons basil – chopped and fresh
- ➢ 3 tablespoons parsley – chopped and fresh (with one tablespoon for garnishing)
- ➢ 1/2 teaspoon salt
- ➢ 4 whole eggs, large and scrambled
- ➢ Black ground pepper – freshly ground

Directions: You will need a large skillet to cook this dish. Begin by heating a tablespoon of the fresh virgin olive oil in the pan. Put in garlic, pepper, and onions in the pan. Stir the food often and allow to sauté for a period of five minutes. Next, add the pepper salt, parsley, and basil. Cook on medium high temperatures for an additional two minutes. Take the mixture and put it on a plate.

Now add the second teaspoon of olive oil to the pan and put the scrambled eggs into the pan for cooking. Make sure the mixture is spread evenly around the surface of the skillet. Cook for three to five minutes, allowing bubbles to form along the edges of the eggs and for the eggs to cook enough to flip them without breakage.

Using a spatula, flip the eggs over in the pan. On one-half of the omelet, add the veggie mix you already cooked and then, with the spatula, fold the uncovered omelet side over on top of the now covered side of the egg omelet.

Place the omelet onto a cutting board or a platter. One-half of the omelet is equal to one serving.

Chapter 9: Dessert

Remember, the Mediterranean diet plan is one where you are not forced to deprive yourself. This means you don't have to feel guilty if you indulge in dessert. Of course, there are desserts that fit right into this super healthy meal plan.

Chilled and Fresh Italian Custard

If you've ever tried gelato than you know the desserts that stem from Italian style cuisine are utterly amazing! Here you can enjoy a delicious, fresh, and healthy version of an Italian Custard, otherwise called *panna cota*. The dessert is light and perfect to follow the larger dinner meal to ensure your hunger remains curbed.

Ingredients (Makes Four Servings)
- ➢ 1 teaspoon - flavorless, sugar-free gelatin
- ➢ 2 tablespoons – heavy cream
- ➢ 3 tablespoons- low-fat milk
- ➢ 2 tablespoons - sugar
- ➢ 2 tablespoons- pure, raw honey – unprocessed
- ➢ 1/3 cup - raspberries
- ➢ 1/3 cup - strawberries
- ➢ 1/3 cup - blackberries
- ➢ 1/4 crushed - walnuts
- ➢ 3/4 cups – heavy cream

Directions: Put 1/4 cup of the heavy cream in a bowl and spread the teaspoon of sugar-free, flavorless gelatin. Set aside for a minute – this will permit the mixture to soften the gelatin powder.

Put the rest of the cream, sugar, and the milk into a pan and boil. Make sure you stir the mixture so it doesn't burn and create curdles in the mix. Once you've got it to reach a boil, take the pan off the heat. Using a fork or a whisk, mix up the gelatin to ensure it is mixed and dissolved well. Set out four custard cups and pour the mix into the cups up to the edge. Put in the fridge and allow to chill for a period of six hours.

When ready to serve, take the mold out of the custard cups and flip onto dessert plates.
Use the honey as a sweet topper – drizzle it over the panna cotta. Top with the berry mix consisting of fresh strawberries, raspberries, and blueberries. Top off with crushed walnuts.

Apple Bake Mediterranean-Style

Baked apples give you the flavor of apple pie without all the calories and carbohydrates that come with it. You also get all the vitamins from this tasty dessert. This treat will leave you satisfied and guilt-free!

Ingredients (Makes Four Servings)
- ➢   1/4 teaspoon - allspice
- ➢   1/4 teaspoon - nutmeg

- ➢ 1/2 cup - yellow raisins
- ➢ 1/2 - lemon, squeezed for the juice
- ➢ 1/2 cup - chopped almonds
- ➢ 1/2 dried - cranberries
- ➢ 1/2 teaspoons - ground cinnamon
- ➢ 4 - medium sized Granny Smith apples
- ➢ 4 tablespoons honey – pure, unprocessed
- ➢ Lemon zest

Directions: Preheat the oven to 350 degrees. The apples for this recipe must be cored, and then you add them to an appropriately sized baking dish. Set the apples aside. In a bowl, mix together the ground cinnamon, dried cranberries, chopped almonds, yellow raisins, nutmeg, and allspice. Also mix in the honey, lemon zest, and ground cinnamon. The cored center is empty in each apple: use the mix to stuff the apples full of the delicious ingredients. Pile on the rest of the mix on top of the stuffed apples and make sure you use it all.

Make sure the baking dish about a half inch of water in the bottom before putting the stuffed apples into the oven. Cook for about 45 minutes until the apples are tender. One apple is equal to one serving. Pour remaining fill over the apples in even distribution. Enjoy!

Conclusion

The Mediterranean diet has proven successful for many people looking to implement a healthy way of eating into their lifestyles. While not a diet that deprives, the Mediterranean food pattern, instead, helps you feel full longer and you are therefore more satisfied. The meals are delicious and loaded with the nutrients your body craves for optimal health. Thus, you can maintain weight or lose weight easily by adhering to the plan, all while remaining satisfied with the foods you are consuming. Even better, this diet promotes socialization and the ritualization of eating, so you begin to treat time times you consume foods as something special or sacred: This means more dedication to considering what you are eating and when you are eating. Essentially, when you treat food consumption as a sacred practice, you begin to recognize the sacredness of your own body and health.

Printed in Great Britain
by Amazon